CRITERIA AND GUIDELINES
FOR THE EVALUATION OF
BACCALAUREATE NURSING PROGRAMS

1991

Pub. No. 15-2474

Council of Baccalaureate and Higher Degree Programs

NATIONAL LEAGUE FOR NURSING • NEW YORK

Copyright ©1992 by
National League for Nursing Press
350 Hudson Street
New York, New York 10014

ISBN O-88737-552-9

Printed in the United States of America

Contents

PREFACE

This document is designed as the 1991 *Criteria and Guidelines for the Evaluation of Baccalaureate and Higher Degree Programs in Nursing* and as a companion manual to the *Policies and Procedures of Accreditation for Programs in Nursing Education*, 6th Edition, 1990. The purposes of the manual are: (1) to foster uniform interpretation of the criteria/outcomes through provision of explicit guidelines, (2) to facilitate development of the Self-Study Report by offering suggestions for evidence to be included in the report and for the format of the report, and (3) to promote efficient and effective accreditation site visits by suggesting materials which should be available for program evaluator review.

PREPARED BY
COUNCIL OF BACCALAUREATE
AND HIGHER DEGREE PROGRAMS

Accreditation Committee
1989–1991

Gloria Donnelly, PhD, RN, FAAN, Chair
David Allen, PhD, RN, FAAN
Kathleen Powers, EdD, RN
Cathleen Shultz, PhD, RN
Ellen Strachota, PhD, RN

SECTION I
OVERVIEW OF NLN ACCREDITATION

As one of four education councils of the National League for Nursing, the Council of Baccalaureate and Higher Degree Programs subscribes to the Philosophy and Purposes of NLN Accreditation set forth in the *Policies and Procedures of NLN Accreditation for Programs in Nursing Education* (6th Edition).

The Philosophy of NLN Accreditation

The NLN Accreditation Program is founded on the belief that specialized accreditation provides for the maintenance and enhancement of educational quality, provides a basic assurance of program improvement, and contributes to the improvement of nursing practice. The achievement of accreditation in nursing indicates to the general public and the educational community that a nursing program has clear and appropriate educational mission and goals and is providing the conditions under which its mission and goals can be fulfilled. Emphasis is placed upon the total nursing program and its compliance with predetermined criteria.

The individuality of the institution in which the nursing program is located is of utmost importance. The NLN believes that the accreditation process focuses on the nursing program within the context of the governing organization's mission and goals and is complementary to regional institutional accreditation. Accreditation activities should be coordinated with other officially recognized regional and specialized accrediting bodies whenever possible.

The paramount beliefs that support the NLN accreditation process are peer evaluation and systematic self-study by the program seeking accreditation. As a voluntary process, accreditation gives to all those concerned a major role.

NLN believes that agency and/or individual members should share in the responsibility for the development of accreditation policies, uniform procedures, council procedures, and evaluation criteria; for participating in accreditation visits; for serving on boards and committees; for initiating changes in the process. Review boards and committees concerned with accreditation should be representative of the profession and the public nursing serves.

As the single designated accrediting agency for nursing education, the NLN subscribes to uniform accreditation policies and procedures among councils and to an organizational mechanism for approval of council variations. NLN values the role of the educational councils in the development of council procedures and evaluation criteria, and in recommending changes in accreditation policies and uniform procedures, and believes the integrity of the councils is to be maintained.

The policies, procedures, and criteria followed by NLN in accrediting educational programs in nursing are based on principles widely accepted and tested in general and professional education. Furthermore, all those involved in the process must be alert to current developments in education and nursing; to the effectiveness of current policies, procedures and criteria; and to the evidence of need for change. A systematic, ongoing evaluation of all components of the accreditation process is essential to ensure an up-to-date and valid accrediting program.

The NLN has achieved documented success as an accrediting agency in the development and maintenance of sound accreditation practices for the benefit of nursing education, the nursing profession, and society. NLN believes that accreditation should remain an activity of private organizations as a non-governmental, voluntary process.

The Purposes of NLN Accreditation

The purposes of accreditation programs in nursing are:

> To foster the continuous development and improvement in quality of educational programs in nursing throughout the United States and its territories.

> To evaluate nursing programs in relation both to their stated purposes and objectives and to the established criteria for accreditation.

> To involve administrators of the governing institutions and the administrators, faculties, and students of nursing programs in the process of continuous self-study and improvement of their programs.

> To bring together practitioners, faculty and students in an activity directed toward improving educational preparation for nursing practice.

> To provide an external peer-review process.

Role of the Councils in the Accreditation Process

The educational councils of the National League for Nursing play a paramount role in the accreditation process in three major ways:

1. Development and approval of the criteria for the evaluation of programs in nursing of the type with which each particular council is concerned.

2. Development and approval of council procedures that facilitate the accreditation process at the council level.

3. Recommending changes in the accreditation policies and the uniform procedures.

SECTION II
PREPARATION OF THE SELF-STUDY REPORT

The Self-Study Process

Purpose

The Council of Baccalaureate and Higher Degree Programs views the process of self-study as both opportunity and responsibility. It is an opportunity for the nursing unit and the governing organization to systematically

- examine the outcomes of its efforts,
- identify strengths and diagnose difficulties, and
- decide on strategies for improvement and maintenance of quality nursing programs.

It is a responsibility of the nursing unit and the governing organization for accountability to students, employers, and recipients of care for providing and maintaining quality nursing educational programs. The data generated by the self-study is used by program evaluators and boards of review to evaluate whether nursing programs meet accreditation criteria.

Participants

Self-study is the combined effort of organizational administrators, nursing unit administrators, faculty, staff, students, and others concerned in the nursing education enterprise.

Process

Self-study process activities that precede the writing of the report are conducted using strategies most useful and facilitative for the participants involved. The self-study process involves the following:

1. Exploration of the beliefs and goals of the program and services of the nursing unit and their congruency with the mission of the governing organization.

2. Assessment of program components considered necessary to achieve outcomes, e.g., structure and governance, evaluation plan, within the context of the mission and goals.

3. Examination of on-going processes designed to maintain and improve all program components.

4. Assessment of outcomes of the nursing unit's programs and operations and their congruency with the nursing unit's mission and goals.

Preparation of the Report

The Self-Study Report is an outcome of the self-study process. It is used by the program evaluators and the Board of Review as one of the primary documents in the evaluation of nursing programs.

The Self-Study Report is completed on the following pages or on the Self-Study Disc (forthcoming). The format is designed to be user friendly. The report, including appendices, should be no longer than 200 pages for Baccalaureate Programs and 250 pages for Baccalaureate and Masters Programs.

Components of the Report

The Self-Study Report is divided into five parts:

1. The Fact Sheet is to provide general information about the governing organization and the nursing unit; numbers and categories of nursing faculty; and current student enrollment by program in the academic term preceding the site visit.

2. Brief Overview of the Program is to provide program evaluators and the Board of Review with general information about the following:

    A. Description of the Governing Organization.

    B. Overview and history of the nursing unit/programs within the governing organization (degrees offered, curriculum tracks in graduate and undergraduate programs, satellite and extension offerings, continuing education courses, research centers and nursing centers), including major developments since the last accreditation review, if applicable.

    C. Demographic description of students and/or learner characteristics.

    D. Composite description of the total faculty in the nursing unit and their activities (Faculty Data Profile - Section VII).

    E. How representative is the information of the current academic term? Are significant differences expected to occur between the writing of the final self-study report and the visit? If yes, explain in a minimum of two pages.

3. Documentation related to criteria 1 through 19, pages 6-31.

    This section of the self-study report provides evidence with respect to criteria (–1 through –19). These criteria relate to those program components considered necessary to produce positive outcomes of the nursing unit's programs and services. The format for reporting evidence on each criterion is as follows:

    A. Each criterion is stated at the top of the page.

    B. Suggested documentation for each criterion is listed and should be included in the space provided for responses (see SECTION V for format).

    C. Evidence that should be available for program evaluators during the site visit is listed in a Table or an Appendix for each. The nursing unit should feel free to provide evidence to evaluators deemed important but not listed.

    D. Definitions of terms specific to each criterion are provided in the glossary (Section IV) to clarify the nature of the evidence to be reported.

4. Documentation related to criterion 20.

    This section of the Self-Study Report provides evidence of outcomes of the nursing unit's programs and services. Reporting is required on outcomes 20.1 THROUGH 20.5. From a menu of 8 optional outcome criteria, reporting is required on two.

    NOTE: Required and optional criteria reflect a grounding in nursing knowledge and replace the process oriented curricular criteria previously used. Faculty may design any curriculum that is consistent with the nursing unit's mission statement (which includes standards of professional nursing) and assists students in meeting these outcomes.

5. Evaluation of the Self-Study Guidelines

    At the end of this report is a form that asks the nursing faculty to evaluate the usefulness of these Guidelines. Please answer the questions and comment in the space provided. Evaluation form is to be completed and added at the end of the self-study. These pages do not count toward the page limitation of the report. Program Evaluators and Board of Review members will also be asked to evaluate guidelines. Sample evaluation forms are included for your information.

These guidelines for preparing the self-study report should be used in conjunction with the following documents:

1. National League for Nursing (1990). *Policies and Procedures of Accreditation for Programs in Nursing Education*, Sixth Edition, New York: NLN

2. Program Evaluators' Report Form

3. Competencies (forthcoming)

SECTION III CRITERIA, GUIDELINES FOR INTERPRETATION AND EVIDENCE

STRUCTURE AND GOVERNANCE

CRITERION 1: The mission and goals of the nursing unit are consistent with those of the governing organization (or differences are explained). They reflect a commitment to a culturally, racially and ethnically diverse community and commitment to a specified set of socially responsible standards of professional nursing.

I. Documentation:

A. Comment in the narrative or in tabular format on the consistency between the nursing unit's and governing organization's mission and goals.

B. Describe how the mission and goals of the governing organization and the nursing unit reflect a commitment to the diversity of the community in which the institution exists.

C. Discuss how the nursing unit's mission and goals are responsive to an identified set of professional nursing standards.

D. Describe how the mission and goals of the organization and nursing unit, as reflected in policies, etc., are implemented to assure a commitment to a diverse community and to professional nursing standards.

E. Describe the results of these efforts.

II. Evidence for Program Evaluators:

A. Self-Study Report

B. Institutional Policies

C. Nursing Policies

D. Mission and Goals

E. Professional Nursing Standards

III. Definitions:

A. Governing organization

B. Nursing unit

C. Mission and goals

D. Professional nursing standards

Note: Refer to Glossary of Terms, Format Guidelines, and Program Evaluators' Evidence Table (SECTIONS IV, V, VI) for preparing this report.

CRITERION 2: Faculty, administrators and students participate in the governance of the organization and the nursing unit in accordance with the opportunities provided by the organizational structure.

I. Documentation:

A. Comment in brief narrative form to what extent faculty, administrators and students participate in and influence the governance of the organization and the nursing unit. Provide diagrams or organizational charts for the following: the governing organization, the administrative unit of the governing organization in which the nursing unit resides, the nursing unit organization and/or its components. (Note: Address all nursing programs and components in the governing organization.)

B. Provide in tabular format evidence of faculty, administrator and student participation in the governance of:

1. governing organization (e.g., past 2 to 5 years)

2. nursing unit (e.g., past 2 to 5 years)

. . .

Suggested Table 2-A
Participation on Committees of Governing Organization

Committee or Council of the Governing Institute	Name of Faculty or Student (Specify)	Term
Univ. Promotion & Tenure	B. Jones (Faculty)	1990-94

. . .

Suggested Table 2-B
Participation on Committees of the Nursing Unit

Committee of the Nursing Unit	Name of Faculty/Student (Specify)	Term
Curriculum Committee (Undergraduate)	S. Smith (Faculty) J. Newell (Student)	1991-94 1990-92

. . .

II. **Evidence for Program Evaluators:**
    A. Committee minutes
    B. Bylaws
    C. Faculty Handbook (organization and nursing unit)
    D. Faculty Governance (policies)
    E. Faculty and Student Interviews

III. **Definitions:**
    A. Governing organization, components
    B. Administrative unit
    C. Nursing programs
    D. Nursing components
    E. Bylaws

CRITERION 3: The nursing unit is administered by a nurse educator who holds a minimum of a master's degree in nursing and an earned doctorate from a regionally accredited institution and has experience in baccalaureate and/or higher degree programs in nursing.

I. **Documentation:**

A. Specify the academic qualifications of the nurse administrator.

B. Describe the nurse administrator's experience in baccalaureate and/or higher degree programs.

II. **Evidence for Program Evaluators:**

A. Nurse administrator's curriculum vita

III. **Definitions:**

A. Nursing unit

B. Academic Nurse Administrator

Note: The phrase "minimum of a master's degree in nursing" means that the administrator must have earned at least one higher degree in nursing at either the masters or doctoral level.

CRITERION 4: The administrator of the nursing unit has the responsibility and authority for planning and allocating resources in accordance with organizational policies and procedures and with nursing faculty involvement. The administrator's work load permits him/her to carry out administrative and leadership activities.

I. **Documentation:**

A. Describe the governing organization's budget process, specifically addressing the nursing administrator's and nursing faculty's involvement. Include the governing organization's process for determining salary on appointment and annual review and advancement.

B. Describe in narrative or tabular form the workload of the nurse administrator.

C. Provide examples of the nurse administrator's leadership and administrative activities relative to the workload.

II. **Evidence for Program Evaluators:**

A. Guidelines for the governing organization's budget process, nursing unit's faculty meeting minutes or other evidence of faculty involvement with the budgetary process, and budget calendar if available.

III. **Definitions:**

A. Budget process

B. Workload

C. Administrative unit

D. Administrative and leadership activities

E. Governing organization

F. Academic Nurse Administrator

MATERIAL RESOURCES

CRITERION 5: The fiscal resources are adequate to support the nursing unit's goals and are commensurate with resources of the organization.

I. Documentation:

A. Comment in brief narrative the nursing unit's assessment of the adequacy and commensurability of its fiscal resources (e.g., include external funding if applicable).

B. Complete the table summarizing the nursing unit's fiscal resources including fiscal and personnel resources.

• • •

Suggested Table 5-A
Budget for Nursing Unit

Categories	Year Prior to Visit	Year of Visit	Projected Budget Year Following Visit
Personnel			
Salary			
Benefits			
Operations			
Capital			
Total			

Suggested Table 5-B
Administrative and Faculty Salaries

Rank	N	Mean Salary	Length of Appointment *	Mean Years of Service	Comparison * * with data source on faculty salaries
Prof.	3	$50,000	10 month	8	54,000
Assoc. Prof.	6				
Asst. Prof.	12				
Instr.	8				
Dean					
Asst. Dean					

* Length of appointment refers to numbers of months of academic appointment, e.g., 9,10,11,12.

* * Use information from one of the following sources and reference the source of comparison such as:

1. NLN Nurse Faculty Socioeconomic Trends.

2. National data on faculty salaries (e.g. ACE, AACN).

3. Regional or state data on faculty salaries.

4. Other selected scales. (Explain choice of scale in footnote to the chart.)

Note: In institutions where salary data is confidential, Table 5-B is made available to program evaluators at time of site visit.

C. Provide evidence that the governing organization is providing the nursing unit with equitable resources.

D. Describe the type and number of support personnel.

E. Describe resources that exist to support faculty development, research, instruction, and/or clinical practice.

II. **Evidence for Program Evaluators:**

A. Faculty files if available.

B. Current budget materials.

C. Interviews with faculty and administration regarding budget and salaries.

III. **Definitions:**

A. Fiscal resources

B. Operations Budget

C. Capital Budget

D. Support personnel

E. Nursing unit

F. Governing organization

CRITERION 6: The physical facilities are adequate for the nursing unit to accomplish its goals.

I. **Documentation:**

A. Give a general description of the physical facilities allocated to the nursing unit at all sites and comment on their adequacy.

II. **Evidence for Program Evaluators:**

A. Tour to evaluate the adequacy of the following:

1. Office space and office equipment for administrators, faculty and staff.

2. Space for instructional activities, e.g., classrooms, conference rooms, learning laboratories, computer laboratories, etc.

3. Storage space for equipment and instructional materials.

4. Facilities and support equipment available for research.

5. Space for non-instructional activities of faculty, staff and students, lounges, meeting rooms, etc.

B. Tour can include library, computer center, study skills center, learning laboratories, and other pertinent learning resource facilities.

III. **Definitions:**

A. Nursing unit

B. Physical facilities

CRITERION 7:   Comprehensive and current library resources and other learning resources are developed with input from nursing faculty, and are available and accessible.

I.   Documentation:

    A.   Library (The emphasis in this criterion is on accessibility to the library and other learning resources.)

        1.   Give a general description of library facilities and access capabilities of the governing organization's library.

        2.   Assess the currency and adequacy of and accessibility to nursing holdings of the library.

        3.   Describe data bases and search capabilities to which students and faculty have access.

    B.   Other Learning Resources

        1.   Give a general description of software and hardware available to students and faculty to support the goals of the nursing unit.

        2.   Describe other learning resources available to support the goals of the nursing unit, e.g. study skills centers, tutoring, counseling, etc.

    C.   Faculty Input

        1.   Describe the mechanisms by which nursing faculty have input into the development and maintenance of the library and other learning resources.

II.   Evidence for Program Evaluators:

    A.   Tour of library, computer center, study skills center, learning laboratories and other pertinent learning resource facilities.

    B.   Library schedules and other learning center schedules.

    C.   Interviews with students, faculty, and personnel in student services and in the library.

    D.   List of the nursing journals.

    E.   List of publishers for which the library maintains blanket orders.

III.   Definitions:

    A.   Data bases

STUDENTS

CRITERION 8:   Student policies of the nursing unit are public, accessible, non-discriminatory and are consistent with the organization. Policies which differ from those of the organization are justified by nursing unit goals.

I.   Documentation:

    A.   List the documents and page numbers where the following policies are published.

        1.   Policies related to non-discrimination

        2.   Admission

        3.   Progression

        4.   Retention

        5.   Dismissal

        6.   Validation and/or articulation

        7.   Graduation

        8.   Grievance and appeal process

    B.   Justify policies that differ from the governing organization's policies.

    C.   Explain the process by which changes in policies are communicated to students.

II.   Evidence for Program Evaluators:

    A.   Policy statements/documents on admission, progression, retention, dismissal, validation and/or articulation, graduation, grievance or other policies not listed but deemed pertinent by the nursing unit.

    B.   Interviews with students, faculty.

    C.   Minutes of meetings showing policy implementation.

    D.   Students files and/or pertinent data such as transcripts, etc.

FACULTY

CRITERION 9: The numbers and utilization of full-time and part-time faculty are appropriate to meet nursing unit goals.

I. Documentation:

A. Complete the Faculty Profile (SECTION VII) for all full and part time faculty during the semester the self-study is completed. This profile may need to be updated at the time of the visit.

B. Describe the type of faculty appointments in the organization and nursing unit.

. . .

Suggested Table 9-A
Full-Time Faculty Profile

Name	Bacc. and Graduate Degrees	Rank	Tenured	Date of Initial Appointment

. . .

Suggested Table 9-B
Part-time Faculty Profile

Name	Bacc. and Graduate Degrees	Rank	Tenured	Date of Initial Appointment

. . .

C. Complete the Faculty Utilization Profile for full- and part-time faculty to reflect the semester the self-study is completed.

. . .

Suggested Table 9-C
Faculty Utilization Profile*

Name	%Teaching/ Advisement	%Admin	%Committee Univ/Dept.	%Scholarly Activity	%Practice	%Service

*   Use categories appropriate to the organization's position descriptions.

Note: Table may be modified to reflect the organization/nursing unit's characteristics, categories, structure, etc.

. . .

D.   Comment on how faculty utilization relates to the mission and goals of the governing organization.

E.   Complete the form that demonstrates Faculty/Student ratios in classroom and in clinical practice.

. . .

Suggested Table 9-D
Faculty/Student Ratios in Classroom

Course	# Sections	Faculty	Faculty/Student ratio

. . .

Suggested Table 9-E
Faculty/Student Ratios in Clinical Practice

Course	# Sections	Faculty	Faculty/Student ratio

. . .

II.   Evidence for Program Evaluators:

    A.   Faculty vitae.

    B.   Faculty files if applicable.

    C.   Faculty interview and visitation of classes and clinical practice areas.

    D.   Class and clinical laboratory schedules and student lists.

    E.   Student interviews.

III.   Definitions:

    A.   Full-time faculty

    B.   Part-time faculty

CRITERION 10: Faculty hold, as a minimum, a master's degree in nursing.* The academic and experiential qualifications and diversity of backgrounds of the faculty are appropriate to their roles and to meet nursing unit goals. Faculty maintain expertise appropriate to their teaching responsibilities.

I. Documentation:

A. Complete the following tables for full- and part-time faculty on the relationship between the academic and experiential preparation of the faculty and their primary focus of teaching responsibilities OR have each faculty member write one comprehensive paragraph on how their academic and experiential qualifications are appropriate to their teaching responsibilities.

. . .

Suggested Table 10.A
Clinical and Role Preparation and Primary Focus
of Teaching Responsibilities for Full-Time Faculty

Name	Degrees	Primary Focus of Teaching	Relevant Clinical Prep	Relevant Role Prep	* * Relevant Other Experience
M. Pearl	MS	Adult Health and Illness	Health Assessment, health promotion	Teaching	
R. Travis	MSN	Psychiatric.	Psychiatric Nursing	Clinical Spec.	

. . .

Suggested Table 10.B
Clinical and Role Preparation and Primary Focus
of Teaching Responsibilities for Part-Time Faculty

Name	Degrees	Primary Focus of Teaching	Relevant Clinical Prep	Relevant Role Prep	* * Relevant Other Experience

* Note: The phrase "minimum of a master's degree in nursing" means that the faculty must have earned at least one higher degree in nursing at either the master's or doctoral level or both.

* * Give an example of relevant other experience (i.e. Faculty Practice, Certification, etc).

. . .

II. Evidence for Program Evaluators:
    A.   Faculty vitae
    B.   Class and clinical laboratory assignments

III. Definitions:
    A.   Full-time faculty
    B.   Part-time faculty

CRITERION 11:   A majority of faculty members currently teaching graduate courses hold earned doctorates from regionally accredited institutions.

I.   Documentation:

A.   In tabular form list graduate courses taught for the semester of the visit, assigned faculty, degrees and institution conferring the doctorate, if applicable.

. . .

Suggested Table 11.A
Overview of Graduate Courses and Faculty

Graduate course Number and title	Faculty	Degrees	Institution conferring doctorate

. . .

II.   Evidence for Program Evaluators:

A.   Faculty vitae

B.   Class schedules

CRITERION 12: Faculty policies of the organization and nursing unit are publicly accessible, non-discriminatory and consistent with each other. Policies of the nursing unit which differ from those of the organization are justified by nursing unit goals.

I. Documentation:

    A. List the documents and page numbers where the following policies are published.

        1. Policies related to non-discrimination

        2. Appointment

        3. Academic rank

        4. Salary and benefits

        5. Rights and responsibilities (including grievance or appeals processes)

        6. Promotion

        7. Tenure

        8. Termination

    B. Justify policies of the nursing organization that differ from the parent organization.

    C. Explain policy differences that may be published in documents.

II. Evidence for Program Evaluators:

    A. Faculty Bylaws

    B. Faculty handbook in which the above listed policies are published

    C. Interviews with faculty

    D. Minutes of meetings showing policy implementation

    E. Faculty files if applicable

III. Definitions:

    A. Governing organization

    B. Nursing unit

CURRICULUM

All Nursing Programs

CRITERION 13: The curriculum for all nursing programs (including master's, where appropriate) are consistent with the mission of the nursing unit.

I. **Documentation:**

    A. Describe the relationship between nursing curricula of all programs and mission of the nursing unit. The term mission can refer to philosophy, frameworks, or a commensurable term used by the nursing unit.

    B. Discuss how the nursing curriculum reflects standards for professional nursing.

II. **Evidence for Program Evaluators:**

    A. Mission and goals of the nursing unit

    B. Complete nursing course syllabi

    C. Sample of student papers and projects

    D. Observation of teaching and learning

III. **Definitions:**

    A. Curricula

    B. Professional nursing standards

Curriculum for Baccalaureate Programs

CRITERION 14: The curriculum focuses on the discipline of nursing and is supported by cognates in the arts, sciences and humanities.

I. Documentation:

    A. Describe the ways in which the curricular focus is on the discipline of nursing and is supported by cognates in the arts, sciences and humanities.

    B. Provide an overview of the total curriculum plans for all programs including cognates in the arts, sciences and/or humanities and all required nursing courses.

II. Evidence for Program Evaluators:

    A. Catalog

    B. Course syllabi

    C. Student files

    D. Minutes of meetings

III. Definitions:

    A. Cognates

    B. Curricula

CRITERION 15:   In baccalaureate programs, the majority of coursework in nursing is at the upper-division level.

I.   Documentation:

A.   Describe the placement of nursing major courses at the upper division.

B.   If applicable, describe rationale and methods for validating prior learning in nursing.

II.   Evidence for Program Evaluators:

A.   Student records

B.   Transfer evaluations

C.   Articulation agreements

D.   Validation tools

E.   Evaluation policies

CRITERION 16: The clinical facilities are adequate and provide opportunities for a variety of learning activities that promote attainment of the objectives of the curriculum.

I.   Documentation:

   A.   Provide in narrative and/or tabular form a comprehensive description and assessment of the adequacy of clinical facilities used in all undergraduate programs.

II.   Evidence for Program Evaluators:

   A.   Visits to clinical facilities

   B.   Affiliation agreements/contracts

III.   Definitions:

   A.   Objectives

Curriculum for the Master's Degree

CRITERION 17:   The master's curriculum builds on the knowledge and competencies of baccalaureate education in nursing and provides for the attainment of advanced knowledge and practice of nursing. It is consistent with the nursing unit's mission.

I.   **Documentation:**

   A.   Describe how the master's curriculum builds on the knowledge and competencies of baccalaureate nursing education and leads to the attainment of advanced knowledge and practice.

   B.   Diagram the total curriculum plan for the master's in nursing program including all tracks.

   C.   Justify any inconsistencies between the master's curriculum and the nursing unit's mission.

II.   **Evidence for the Program Evaluators:**

   A.   Catalog

   B.   Complete course syllabi

   C.   Student files

   D.   Minutes of meetings

III.   **Definitions:**

   A.   Curricula

   B.   Nursing unit

   C.   Mission

CRITERION 18: The facilities for practica are adequate and provide opportunities for a variety of learning activities that promote attainment of curriculum objectives.

I. Documentation:

A. Provide a comprehensive description and assessment of the adequacy of clinical facilities used in all graduate programs.

II. Evidence for Program Evaluators:

A. Visits to clinical facilities

B. Affiliation agreements/contracts.

III. Definitions:

A. Objectives

Evaluation

CRITERION 19: There is ongoing systematic evaluation of all program components which is used for development, maintenance and revision of the program.

I. **Documentation:**

   A. In narrative or tabular form describe the nursing unit's master plan of evaluation for all program components.

   B. Give examples of how evaluation data were used to develop, maintain or revise a component or components of the program.

II. **Evidence for Program Evaluators:**

   A. Annual reports

   B. Meeting minutes

   C. Interviews with administrators, faculty, and students that validate implementation of the master plan of evaluation.

III. **Definitions:**

   A. Program components

CRITERION 20: The evaluation plan includes the required and selected optional outcome criteria which follow. All outcomes should be consistent with the mission of the unit.

REQUIRED OUTCOME CRITERIA
FOR EACH PROGRAM UNDER REVIEW

There are five (5) required outcome criteria: (1) critical thinking, (2) communication, (3) therapeutic nursing interventions, (4) graduation rates, and (5) employment rates. Required outcomes are to be reported for each program under review. Required outcomes may be defined differently for each program. For master's programs, required outcomes need not be reported for each track but for the total program.

REQUIRED OUTCOME CRITERION 1: Critical Thinking

This outcome reflects students' skills in reasoning, analysis, research, or decision making relevant to the discipline of nursing.

I.   Documentation:

    A.   Give the nursing unit's definition of critical thinking appropriate to each nursing program.

    B.   Provide a rationale and assessment of the methods or processes used to evaluate or measure critical thinking.

    C.   Report critical thinking outcome data and its use in the development, maintenance and revision of program/s.

II.   Evidence for Program Evaluators:

    A.   Reports

    B.   Committee minutes

    C.   Measurement instruments.

III. Definitions:

    A.   Nursing unit

    B.   Mission

    C.   Outcomes

REQUIRED OUTCOME CRITERION 2: Communication

This outcome reflects students' abilities in areas such as written, oral and nonverbal communication, group process, information technology and/or media production.

I. **Documentation:**

A. Give the nursing unit's definition of communication abilities appropriate to each nursing program.

B. Provide a rationale and assessment of the methods or processes used to evaluate or measure communication abilities.

C. Report communication ability outcome data and their use in the development, maintenance and revision of the program.

II. **Evidence for Program Evaluators:**

A. Reports

B. Committee minutes

C. Measurement instruments

III. **Definitions:**

A. Nursing Unit

B. Mission

C. Outcomes

REQUIRED OUTCOME CRITERION 3: Therapeutic Nursing Interventions

This outcome reflects students' abilities to perform theory-based nursing interventions including psychomotor and psychosocial therapeutics directed at individuals and/or aggregates.

I. **Documentation:**

   A. Give the nursing unit's definition of therapeutic nursing interventions abilities appropriate to each program under review.

   B. Provide a rationale and assessment of the methods or processes used to evaluate therapeutic nursing intervention abilities.

   C. Report therapeutic nursing intervention abilities outcome data and their use in the development, maintenance and revision of the program/s.

II. **Evidence for Program Evaluators:**

   A. Reports

   B. Committee minutes

   C. Measurement instruments

III. **Definitions:**

   A. Nursing Unit

   B. Mission

   C. Outcomes

REQUIRED OUTCOME CRITERION 4: Graduation Rates

This outcome reflects numbers of students entering, length of time in program and numbers graduated. Other issues could include "stop outs" or criteria used to identify "at risk students."

I.   **Documentation:**

    A.   Report the number of students that have been admitted to and graduated from the program/s and the average length of time from admission to graduation. Specify the time frame within which this data is being reported.

    B.   Specify at what point students are considered admitted to the nursing major (e.g., freshman year, etc.).

II. **Evidence for Program Evaluators:**

    A.   Reports

    B.   Committee minutes

    C.   Measurement instruments

III. **Definitions:**

    A.   Nursing Unit

    B.   Mission

    C.   Outcomes

REQUIRED OUTCOME CRITERION 5: Patterns of Employment

This outcome reflects employment patterns of graduates. The purpose is to document both initial employment and changes in employment over time.

I. **Documentation:**

A. Provide a rationale and assessment of instruments/methods with which employment patterns of graduates of programs are surveyed and time periods of surveys.

B. Report outcome data on employment patterns of graduates of each program under review upon graduation and at a time interval/s specified by the nursing unit.

II. **Evidence for Program Evaluators:**

A. Reports

B. Committee minutes

C. Measurement instruments

III. **Definitions:**

A. Nursing Unit

B. Mission

C. Outcomes

OPTIONAL OUTCOME CRITERIA

There are eight (8) optional outcome criteria: (1) program satisfaction, (2) professional development, (3) personal development, (4) attainment of credentials, (5) organization or work environment, (6) scholarship, (7) service, and (8) nursing unit defined. Select two of the eight optional outcomes for each program under review, that best reflects the unique mission of the nursing unit within the context of the governing organization. For master's programs optional outcomes need not be reported for each track but for the graduate program as a whole.

OPTIONAL OUTCOME CRITERION 1: Program Satisfaction

This outcome reflects the satisfaction level or evaluation of the program by major constituencies such as students, alumni, employers or faculty.

I. **Documentation:**

   A. Give the nursing unit's definition of program satisfaction and the target group/s for the evaluation.

   B. Describe how the reporting of this outcome reflects the nursing unit's mission within the context of the governing organization.

   C. Provide a rationale and assessment of the methods or processes used to evaluate Program Satisfaction.

   D. Report Program Satisfaction outcome data and their use in the development, maintenance and revision of the program/s.

II. **Evidence for Program Evaluators:**

   A. Reports

   B. Committee minutes

   C. Measurement instruments

III. **Definitions:**

   A. Nursing Unit

   B. Mission

   C. Outcomes

OPTIONAL OUTCOME CRITERION 2: Professional development

This outcome reflects the graduates' participation in professional activities such as continuing education, formal education, professional organizations and research.

I. **Documentation:**

A. Give the nursing unit's definition of professional development and the target group/s for the evaluation.

B. Describe how the reporting of this outcome reflects the nursing unit's mission within the context of the governing organization.

C. Provide a rationale and assessment of the methods or processes used to evaluate professional development.

D. Report professional development outcome data and their use in the development, maintenance and revision of the program/s.

II. **Evidence for Program Evaluators:**

A. Reports

B. Committee minutes

C. Measurement instruments

III. **Definitions:**

A. Nursing Unit

B. Mission

C. Outcomes

OPTIONAL OUTCOME CRITERION 3: Personal Development

This outcome reflects aspects of graduates' personal development with respect to program support of students' mental and physical health, health promoting activities, self esteem, self efficacy, pursuit of life-long learning and involvement as citizens.

I. **Documentation:**

   A. Give the nursing unit's definition of personal development and the target group/s for the evaluation.

   B. Describe how the reporting of this outcome reflects the nursing unit's mission within the context of the governing organization.

   C. Provide a rationale and assessment of methods or processes used to evaluate personal development.

   D. Report personal development outcome data and their use in the development, maintenance and revision of the program/s.

II. **Evidence for Program Evaluators:**

   A. Reports

   B. Committee minutes

   C. Measurement instruments

III. **Definitions:**

   A. Nursing Unit

   B. Mission

   C. Outcomes

This outcome reflects attainment of credentials that are relevant to the unit's mission. This could include passing certification examinations or other tests appropriate to the unit's mission.

I. Documentation:

   A. Give the nursing unit's definition of credentials, e.g. licensure, certifications, and advanced degrees; and the target group/s for the evaluation.

   B. Describe how the reporting of this outcome reflects the nursing unit's mission within the context of the governing organization.

   C. Provide a rationale and assessment of the methods or processes used to evaluate attainment of credentials.

   D. Report attainment of credentials outcome data and their use in the development, maintenance and revision of the program/s.

II. Evidence for Program Evaluators:

   A. Reports

   B. Committee minutes

   C. Measurement instruments

III. Definitions:

   A. Nursing Unit

   B. Mission

   C. Outcomes

OPTIONAL OUTCOME CRITERION 5: Organization or Work Environment

This outcome reflects the extent to which the organization supports faculty and staff well being. Examples could include job satisfaction, mental and physical health, and organizational commitment.

I.   Documentation:

   A.   Give the nursing unit's definition of organization or work environment variables and the target group/s for the evaluation.

   B.   Describe how the reporting of this outcome reflects the nursing unit's mission within the context of the governing organization.

   C.   Provide a rationale and assessment of the methods or processes used to evaluate variables related to organization or work environment.

   D.   Report organization or work environment outcome data and their use in the development, maintenance and revision of the program/s.

II. Evidence for Program Evaluators:

   A.   Reports

   B.   Committee minutes

   C.   Measurement instruments

III. Definitions:

   A.   Nursing Unit

   B.   Mission

   C.   Outcomes

This outcome reflects the generation or dissemination of knowledge through publications, presentations, media, technology or grant writing. Students, faculty and staff * could be seen as contributing to this outcome.

I. **Documentation:**

    A. Give the nursing unit's definition of variables related to scholarship and the target group/s for the evaluation.

    B. Describe how the reporting of this outcome best reflects the nursing unit's mission within the context of the governing organization.

    C. Provide a rationale and assessment of methods or processes used to evaluate variables related to scholarship.

    D. Report scholarship outcome data and its use in the development, maintenance and revision of the program/s.

II. **Evidence for Program Evaluators:**

    A. Reports

    B. Committee minutes

    C. Measurement instruments

III. **Definitions:**

    A. Nursing Unit

    B. Mission

    C. Outcomes

* *Staff* refers to professional staff

OPTIONAL OUTCOME CRITERION 7: Service

This outcome reflects staff, faculty and student participation in activities such as clinical practice, political activism, committees or boards both within the college and in the community.

I.   **Documentation:**

A.   Give the nursing unit's definition of variables related to service and the target group/s for the evaluation.

B.   Describe how the reporting of this outcome best reflects the nursing unit's mission within the context of the governing organization.

C.   Provide a rationale and assessment of methods or processes used to evaluate variables related to service.

D.   Report service outcome data and their use in the development, maintenance and revision of the program/s.

II. **Evidence for Program Evaluators:**

A.   Reports

B.   Committee minutes

C.   Measurement instruments

III. **Definitions:**

A.   Nursing Unit

B.   Mission

C.   Outcomes

OPTIONAL OUTCOME CRITERION 8: Nursing Unit Defined

This is a mission-relevant outcome selected by a program. It would permit the unit to highlight and demonstrate outcomes unique to the nursing unit that are not addressed by previously defined required and optional outcome criteria.

I.   Documentation:

A.   Define the outcome selected by the nursing unit.

B.   Describe how the reporting of this nursing unit defined outcome best reflects the nursing unit's mission within the context of the governing organization.

C.   Provide a rationale and assessment of methods or processes used to evaluate variables related to the nursing unit's defined outcome.

D.   Report outcome data on the nursing unit's defined outcome and its use in the development, maintenance and revision of the programs.

II. Evidence for Program Evaluators:

A.   Reports

B.   Committee minutes

C.   Measurement instruments

III. Definitions:

A.   Nursing Unit

B.   Mission

C.   Outcomes

SECTION IV
GLOSSARY OF TERMS

NLN
Council of Baccalaureate and Higher Degree Programs
Self-Study Guidelines

Academic nurse administrator

The appropriately credentialed nurse educator responsible for the administration of all nursing programs in the governing organization, e.g. Dean, Chair, Director, etc.

Administrative unit

The administrative unit or units within the governing organization in which the department, school resides. Nursing programs may be located in more than one administrative unit.

Administrative and leadership activities

Any internal or external activities other than teaching carried out by the academic nurse administrator/s for purposes of planning, directing, coordinating, improving, or governing within the nursing unit, the academic unit, the governing organization or a professional organization external to the governing organization.

Budget process

Those activities and persons involved over a specified time period (e.g. budget calendar) in development, negotiation, and final approval, and administration of the budget/s for the nursing unit.

Bylaws

Established rules that govern the internal affairs of the organizational entity.

Capital budget

That portion of the nursing unit's budget used for the purchase of items and expenditures that are to be capitalized, e.g., recorded in plant funds. Capitalized assets usually represent an investment of funds with a minimum as defined by the governing organization and ordinarily non-consumable with a useful life line of at least 4 years.

Cognates

Non-nursing courses which are foundational and/or related to the nursing courses in the program/s under review.

Curricula

All courses and planned program activities designated for completing the bachelor's and/or master's degree in nursing.

Data base

A printed or computerized file of library collections, standardized in format and content and organized into interrelated topics or themes.

Fiscal resources

Those resources allocated by the governing organization to the nursing unit to underwrite operation of nursing programs and components.

Full-time faculty

All persons who teach nursing courses in the program/s being reviewed for accreditation status and who have full-time faculty employment status as determined by the governing organization.

Goals

Desired outcomes of the programs of the governing organization and/or nursing unit in general.

Governing organization

The university, college or other organization of which the nursing program is an integral part and which includes shared responsibility for general educational and administrative policy, long range planning, allocation of resources and determination of faculty status.

Mission

The statement approved by the highest authority of the governing organization that provides direction for the programs and services of the institution. The nursing unit may use a term other than mission to title the statements of purpose and direction.

Nursing components

All non-curricular components of nursing programs such as research centers, nursing centers or any other parts of the total program effort.

Nursing program

Plans of study leading to a bachelor's or master's degree in nursing.

Nursing unit

The department, school, division, or college within a governing organization that offers one or more nursing program/s.

Objectives

Assessable outcomes of the instructional process.

Operations budget

That portion of the nursing unit's budget that funds the usual supplies and services needed to operate nursing programs and components within the nursing unit.

Outcomes

Outcomes are performance indicators. As the end product of any activity, outcomes evidence to what extent the purposes of the activity are being achieved. According to Hart and Waltz (1988), "outcomes can be broadly defined as the outputs or results of the program or the activities of the provider."

Part-time faculty

All persons who teach nursing courses in the programs being reviewed for accreditation status and have part-time faculty status as determined by the governing organization. Such faculty may be employed by other agencies and hold primary responsibility for teaching nursing courses by mutual agreement between the governing organization and the agency.

Professional nursing standards

An authoritative set of guidelines approved by nursing faculty for use in the evaluation of professional nursing practice.

Program components

Refers to structure and governance, material resources, students, faculty, curriculum and evaluation.

Salary on annual review and/or advancement

A contracted amount of money granted at times (e.g. once per year, etc.) specified by the governing organization or following an employee performance review (e.g. evaluation) at designated intervals, a promotion in rank or a change in employment responsibilities.

Support personnel

Persons filling authorized salaried positions in the nursing unit whose primary responsibilities include administrative, clerical or other functions other than instruction or educational administration.

Workload

The delineation of contractual responsibilities in hours or time units defined by the governing organization for faculty and administrators.

SECTION V
RECOMMENDATIONS FOR FORMAT

Double spaced

10 or 12 point type (not script)

letter quality (not dot-matrix)

200 pages total for baccalaureate programs, numbered sequentially and including appendices and all documentation.

250 pages total for baccalaureate and master's program.

Documentation and narrative responses must be limited to the space provided or inserted as directed by the Guidelines.

Margins: 1.0 inch top and bottom; 1.5 inch left; .5 inch right.

Bound

15 copies

Completed Guideline Evaluation Form to be included at the end of the Self-Study Report.

All self-study reports and related materials are to be in English.

SECTION VI
RECOMMENDED EVIDENCE
FOR REVIEW BY PROGRAM EVALUATORS

The following evidence is recommended for the designated criteria. The nursing unit should feel free to provide additional evidence to evaluators which is deemed important but not indicated on the list.

Evidence	Criterion																			
	1	2	3	4	5	6	7	8	9	10	11	12	13	14	15	16	17	18	19	20
Governing organization's mission and goal statement	X	-	-	-	-	-	-	-	-	-	-	-	-	-	-	-	-	-	-	-
Nursing unit's mission and goal statement	X	-	-	-	-	-	-	-	-	-	-	-	X	-	-	-	-	-	-	-
Professional nursing standards	X	-	-	-	-	-	-	-	-	-	-	-	X	-	-	-	-	-	-	-
Diagram of governing unit's organizational chart	-	X	-	-	-	-	-	-	-	-	-	-	-	-	-	-	-	-	-	-
Diagram of academic unit's organizational chart	-	X	-	-	-	-	-	-	-	-	-	-	-	-	-	-	-	-	-	-
Diagram of nursing unit's organizational chart	-	X	-	-	-	-	-	-	-	-	-	-	-	-	-	-	-	-	-	-
Committee minutes	-	X	-	X	-	-	X	X	-	-	-	X	X	X	-	-	X	-	X	X
Interviews	X	X	X	X	X	X	X	X	X	X	X	X	X	X	X	X	X	X	X	X
By-laws	-	X	-	-	-	-	-	-	-	-	-	X	-	-	-	-	-	-	-	-
Faculty files (if applicable)	-	-	-	-	X	-	-	-	X	-	X	X	-	-	-	-	-	-	-	-
Curriculum vita of nursing administrator	-	-	X	-	-	-	-	-	-	-	-	-	-	-	-	-	-	-	-	-

Evidence	\multicolumn{20}{c}{Criterion}

Evidence	1	2	3	4	5	6	7	8	9	10	11	12	13	14	15	16	17	18	19	20
Curriculum vita of faculty	-	-	-	-	-	-	-	-	X	X	X	-	-	-	-	-	-	-	-	-
Governing organization's budget process	-	-	-	X	X	-	-	-	-	-	-	-	-	-	-	-	-	-	-	-
Documentation of involvement by faculty, administrators or students	-	X	-	X	-	-	X	-	-	-	-	-	-	-	-	-	-	-	-	-
Budget calendar (if applicable)	-	-	-	X	-	-	-	-	-	-	-	-	-	-	-	-	-	-	-	-
Current budget materials (e.g. computer print-outs etc.)	-	-	-	-	X	-	-	-	-	-	-	-	-	-	-	-	-	-	-	-
Tour of physical facilities allocated to nursing unit	-	-	-	-	-	X	-	-	-	-	-	-	-	-	-	-	-	-	-	-
Tour of library and other learning resources	-	-	-	-	-	-	X	-	-	-	-	-	-	-	-	-	-	-	-	-
Library and other learning resources schedules	-	-	-	-	-	-	X	-	-	-	-	-	-	-	-	-	-	-	-	-
Documents which have published policies	-	-	-	-	-	-	-	X	-	-	-	-	X	-	-	-	-	-	-	-
Visit to classes and/or clinical practice areas	-	-	-	-	-	-	-	-	X	-	-	-	X	X	-	X	-	X	-	-
Class and clinical course schedules	-	-	-	-	-	-	-	-	X	-	-	-	-	X	-	X	-	X	-	-

Evidence	Criterion																			
	1	2	3	4	5	6	7	8	9	10	11	12	13	14	15	16	17	18	19	20
Complete syllabi for each nursing course	-	-	-	-	-	-	-	-	-	-	-	-	X	X	-	-	X	-	-	-
Sample student papers, tests and projects per course	-	-	-	-	-	-	-	-	-	-	-	-	X	-	-	-	X	-	-	-
Catalog	-	-	-	-	-	-	-	-	-	-	-	-	X	X	-	-	X	-	-	-
Curriculum plan overview	-	-	-	-	-	-	-	-	-	-	-	-	X	X	-	-	-	-	-	-
Student records	-	-	-	-	-	-	-	X	-	-	-	-	-	X	X	-	X	-	-	-
Articulation Agreement (if applicable)	-	-	-	-	-	-	-	-	-	-	-	-	-	-	X	-	-	-	-	-
Validating tools and policies	-	-	-	-	-	-	-	X	-	-	-	-	-	-	X	-	-	-	-	-
Affiliation agreements/ contracts	-	-	-	-	-	-	-	-	-	-	-	-	-	-	-	X	-	X	-	-
Nursing unit's annual reports	-	-	-	-	-	-	-	-	-	-	-	-	-	-	-	-	-	-	X	X
Evaluation data results	-	-	-	-	-	-	-	-	-	-	-	-	-	-	-	-	-	-	X	X
Measurement instruments	-	-	-	-	-	-	-	-	-	-	-	-	-	-	-	-	-	-	-	X

SECTION VII
FACULTY PROFILE FORM

FACULTY PROFILE FORM

NAME OF COLLEGE/UNIVERSITY _____

FT/PT & *	Faculty	Date of Initial App't	Rank/ Tenure (T)	Bacc. & Graduate Degrees	Institution Granting Degree	Academic Clinical	Preparation Functional	Course and Area of Responsibility

* faculty teaching nursing courses

FACULTY PROFILE FORM

NAME OF COLLEGE/UNIVERSITY _____

FT/PT & *	Faculty	Date of Initial App't	Rank/ Tenure (T)	Bacc. & Graduate Degrees	Institution Granting Degree	Academic Clinical	Preparation Functional	Course and Area of Responsibility

* faculty teaching nursing courses

SECTION VIII
OUTCOMES BIBLIOGRAPHY

Adair, S. M. (1990, March). Educational outcomes: Their impact on graduate pediatric dentistry education. *Journal of Dental Education, 53*(3), 188–190.

Altieri, G. (1990, Spring). A structural model for student outcomes: Assessment programs in community colleges. *Community College Review, 17*(4), 15–21.

Aper, J. P., et al. (1990, December). Coming to terms with the accountability versus improvement debate in assessment. *Higher Education, 20*(4), 471–483.

Ashcroft, J. (1986, November). Does a degree tell us what a student has learned? *Phi Delta Kappa, 68*(4), 225–227.

Astin, A. W. (1987, Fall). Assessment, value-added, and educational excellence. Student outcomes assessment: What institutions stand to gain. *New Directions for Higher Education* (No. 59, 15(3), 89–107).

Astin, A. W., & Ayala, F. (1987, Summer). Institutional strategies: A consortial approach to assessment. *Educational Record, 68*(3), 47–51.

Baird, L. L. (1988). A map of postsecondary assessment. *Research in Higher Education, 28*(2), 99–115.

Banta, T. W., & Fisher, H. S. (1990, October). An international perspective on assessing baccalaureate program outcomes. *Evaluation Practice, 11*(3), 167–175.

Banta, T. W., & Pike, G. R. (1989, October). Methods for comparing outcomes assessment instruments. *Research in Higher Education, 30*(5), 455–469.

Banta, T. W., et al. (1986, November). Assessment of institutional effectiveness at the University of Tennessee, Knoxville. *International Journal of Institutional Management in Higher Education, 10*(3), 262–271.

Casamassimo, P. S. (1990, March). Assessment of educational outcomes in pediatric dentistry: A site examiner's perspective. *Journal of Dental Education, 53*(3), 191–193.

Chalmers, R. K., et al. (1988, Winter). Assessing the outcomes of pharmacy education—The 1988 Argus commission report. *American Journal of Pharmaceutical Education, 52*(4), 405–408.

Claxton, C., et al. (1987, September–October). Outcomes assessment. *AGB Reports, 29*(5), 32–35.

Cullen, C. L. (1990, March). Defining and assessing affective outcomes in undergraduate pediatric dentistry. *Journal of Dental Education, 53*(3), 184–187.

Denham, C. (1988, Spring). Student outcomes assessment in higher education. *Teacher Education Quarterly, 15*(2), 82–89.

Dennison, G., & Bunda, M. A. (1989, Fall). Assessment and academic judgments in higher education. Achieving assessment goals using evaluation techniques. *New Directions for Higher Education* (No. 67, 17(3), 51–70).

Edwards, D. E., & Brannen, D. E. (1990, February). Current status of outcomes assessment at the MBA level. *Journal of Education for Business, 65*(5), 206–212.

Faughn, J. R., et al. (1990, August). Ensuring quality through outcomes assessment. *Career Training, 7*(1), 12–18.

Frank, J. (1989, Summer). Outcomes assessment: Past, present and future. *Campus Activities Programming, 22*(2), 38–42.

Garcia, M. (1990, Spring). Assessing program effectiveness in an institution with a diverse student body. The effect of assessment on minority student participation. *New Directions for Institutional Research* (No. 65, 17(1), 69–76).

Halpern, D. F. (1987, Fall). Student outcomes assessment: Introduction and overview. Student outcomes assessment: What institutions stand to gain. *New Directions for Higher Education* (No. 59, 15(3), 5–8.).

Hanson, G. R. (1988, Fall). Critical issues in the assessment of value added in education. Implementing outcomes assessment: Promise and perils. *New Directions for Institutional Research* (No. 59, 15(3), 53–67).

Jennings, E. T., Jr. (1989, September–October). Accountability, program quality, outcomes assessment, and graduate education for public affairs and administration. *Public Administration Review, 49*(5), 438–446.

Kassebaum, D. G. (1990, May). The measurement of outcomes in the assessment of educational program effectiveness. *Academic Medicine, 65*(5), 293–296.

Kerschner, L. (1987, Fall). Outcomes assessment in the California master plan. Student outcomes assessment: What institutions stand to gain. *New Directions for Higher Education* (No. 59, 15(3), 29–31).

Kozloff, J. (1987, September). A student-centered approach to accountability and assessment. *Journal of College Student Personnel, 28*(5), 419–424.

Laff, N. S. (1989, Fall). Adventures in the gray zone: Critical & creative thinking and how to structure the personal meaning of education. *Research and Teaching in Developmental Education, 6*(1), 5–20.

Lenburg, C. B., & Mitchell, C. A. (1991, February). Assessment of outcomes: The design and use of real and simulation nursing performance examinations. *Nursing & Health Care, 12*(2), 68–74.

Lenning, O. T. (1988, Fall). Use of noncognitive measures in assessment. Implementing outcomes assessment: Promise and perils. (No. 59, 15(3), 41–52).

Lincoln, Y. S. (1990, February). Program review, accreditation processes, and outcomes assessment: Pressures on institutions of higher education. *Evaluation Practice, 11*(1), 13–23.

Loacker, G. (1988, Summer). Faculty as a force to improve instruction through assessment. Assessing students' learning. *New Directions for Teaching and Learning* (34) 19–32.

McClain, C. J., et al. (1986, November). Northeast Missouri State University's value-added assessment program: A model for educational accountability. *International Journal of Institutional Management in Higher Education, 10*(3), 252–261.

Morganstein, W. M. (1990, June). Outcome measures in dental education—We've only just begun. *Journal of Dental Education, 54*(6), 308–310.

Nichols, J. O., & Wolff, L. A. (1990, Summer). Organizing effective institutional research office. *New Directions for Institutional Research* (No. 66, 17(2), 82–92).

Oakes, J. (1989, Summer). What educational indicators? The case for assessing the school context. *Educational Evaluation and Policy Analysis, 11*(2), 181–199.

Ory, J. C., & Parker, S. A. (1989, August). Assessment activities at large, research universities. *Research in Higher Education, 30*(4), 375–385.

Osigweh, C. A. B. (1986, Summer). An evaluation model of training outcomes for higher education. *Educational Evaluation and Policy Analysis, 8*(2), 167–178.

Osigweh, C. A. B. (1986, Winter). A "value-added" model of measuring performance. *College Teaching, 34*(1), 28–33.

Resnick, D. P., & Goulden, M. (1987, Fall). Assessment, curriculum, and expansion: A historical perspective. Student outcomes assessment: What institutions stand to gain. *New Directions for Higher Education* (No. 59, 15(3), 77–88).

Rogers, B. H., & Gentemann, K. M. (1989, June). The value of institutional research in the assessment of institutional effectiveness. *Research in Higher Education, 30*(3), 345–355.

Spangehl, S. D. (1987, January–February). The push to assess: Why it's feared and how to respond. *Change, 19*(1), 35–39.

Tan, D. L. (1986). The assessment of quality in higher education: A critical review of the literature and research. *Research in Higher Education, 24*(3), 223–265.

Terenzini, P. T. (1989, November–December). Assessment with open eyes: Pitfalls in studying student outcomes. *Journal of Higher Education, 60*(6), 644–664.

Warren, J. (1988, Fall). Cognitive measures in assessing learning. Implementing outcomes assessment: Promise and perils. *New Directions for Institutional Research* (No. 59, 15(3), 29–39).

Williams, D. D. (1986, June). When is naturalistic evaluation appropriate? *New Directions for Program Evaluation, 30*, 85–92.

SECTION IX
EVALUATION

(To be completed by Nursing Unit, Program Evaluators, and Board of Review Members)

INTRODUCTION:

The Baccalaureate and Higher Degree Accreditation Subcommittee is committed to gathering information about the new criteria and guidelines. We are asking nursing units, program evaluators and the Board of Review members to respond to questionnaires. The results will be analyzed and reported for discussion, feedback and revision at the annual Council meeting. Results will be used to further refine the Self-Study Guidelines.

Questions for Nursing Units

1. The Self-Study Guidelines were (circle best response):

too specific	somewhat specific	about right	somewhat general	too general
1	2	3	4	5

too rigid	somewhat rigid	about right	somewhat flexible	too flexible
1	2	3	4	5

prohibits creativity	somewhat prohibits creativity	somewhat facilitated creativity	facilitated creativity	greatly facilitated creativity
1	2	3	4	5

very unclear	somewhat unclear	somewhat clear	clear	extremely clear
1	2	3	4	5

very redundant	somewhat redundant	fairly redundant	a little redundant	not at all redundant
1	2	3	4	5

very hard to follow	somewhat hard to follow	fairly hard to follow	easy to follow	extremely easy to follow
1	2	3	4	5

2. The Guidelines should be closely matched to the Criteria so that the questions asked and documentation required directly address the extent to which the programs met the respective criteria. To what extent did this occur:

never matched	sometimes matched	moderately matched	very often matched	extremely well matched

3. The Self-Study should help a unit identify its strengths and limitations and permit the unit to represent an accurate, complete picture of itself to the program evaluators and the Board of Review. To what extent was this true:

A)   Identified program's strengths:

never occurred	sometimes occurred	moderately occurred	occurred very often	occurred at all times
1	2	3	4	5

B)   Identified program's limitations:

never occurred	sometimes occurred	moderately occurred	occurred very often	occurred at all times
1	2	3	4	5

C)   Produced an accurate and complete picture of program.

not at all true	somewhat true	fairly true	very true	completely true
1	2	3	4	5

Comments:

4. One of the newest features of this set of Criteria and Guidelines is the inclusion of Outcome Criteria. Hence we are especially interested in your experience in addressing Outcome Criteria:

A)   Were practical instruments or measurement processes available?

Yes

No (please comment):

B)   Were the data related to outcomes helpful?

      Yes

      No (please comment)

5.   Does the data related to outcomes have the potential to be helpful for program planning/revision in the future?

      Yes

      No (please comment)

6.   Did you use the resources related to outcomes that were provided in the Guidelines?

      Yes   No

      If yes, were they helpful?

7.   Were the suggestions for preparing for evaluators helpful?

      Yes

      No (please comment):

8. Were the definitions provided in the glossary of terms clear and helpful?

Not at all	Somewhat	Fairly	Quite	Extremely
1	2	3	4	5

If not clear, which need more information?

9. The accreditation and self-study process and procedure often play a role in helping a unit negotiate with the governing organization for resources. To what extent was this true (or will this be true) for your unit?

Not at all true	Not very true	Somewhat true	True	Very True
1	2	3	4	5

10. The evaluators were familiar with the Criteria and Guidelines:

Yes

No (if no, please give examples)

11. The evaluators interpreted the Criteria and Guidelines the same way you did:

Yes

No (if no, please give examples)

12. The evaluators asked only for data that was required by the Guidelines:

    Yes

    No (if no, please give examples)

13. The 200 page limitation on the length of the Self-Study was:

Entirely too short	Too short	About right	Too long	Entirely too long
1	2	3	4	5

    Comment on the length:

14. How difficult was it to provide the data required by the Guidelines?

Much too difficult	Too difficult	Fairly easy	Easy	Extremely easy
1	2	3	4	5

Questions For Program Evaluators

1. Did the general assessment or impression of the program produced by the Self-Study Guidelines correlate well with what you found during your visit?

Not at all	Not very well	Fairly well	Very well	Extremely well
1	2	3	4	5

If not, are there changes in the Guidelines you can suggest that would help?

2. Did the Self-Study Guidelines help you maintain an open-minded, objective approach to your evaluation?

Yes

No

Comment:

3. One goal with the new Guidelines was to produce enough relevant data but not an overwhelming amount of detail. To what extent was this accomplished?

Way too much detail	Too much detail	About the right amount	Not enough detail	Far to little detail
1	2	3	4	5

4. Was there additional information you needed that was not requested in the Guidelines?

Yes

No

Comment:

5. Was information required that you would suggest we delete?

    No

    Yes (please give examples)

6. Another goal was to reduce the report's redundancy without overburdening evaluators. How well was this goal met?

Not at all met	Somewhat met	Fairly well met	Well met	Completely met
1	2	3	4	5

7. How easy was it to achieve reliability to intersubjective agreement (among program evaluators, between evaluators and the unit) on the criteria?

Could not achieve	Somewhat achieved	Fairly achieved	Achieved well	Completely achieved
1	2	3	4	5

8. On the Guidelines?

1	2	3	4	5

9. Please comment on where you had the most difficulty with the criteria and guidelines.

10. Were the definitions clear and helpful?

    Yes

    No

    Comment:

11. Were there other definitions you would like to see added?

Yes

No

Comment:

12. Another goal was to balance the information provided in advance by the self-study with evidence available to program evaluator.

How well was this achieved? (too much in self-study, too much to process on site)

Not at all	Somewhat	Fairly well	Very well	Completely
1	2	3	4	5

13. The major purpose of the Self-Study Guidelines is to facilitate your evaluation of the programs. How well did they do this?

Not at all	Somewhat	Fairly well	Quite well	Extremely well
1	2	3	4	5

14. Did you think the "Suggestions for Preparing for Evaluators" helped the unit prepare for your arrival and review?

Yes

No

Comment:

15. Did the suggestions help you?

Yes

No

Comment:

16. Did the Evaluators' Report Form correlate well with the Guidelines and Criteria:
Yes
No (please give examples)

17. Are there suggestions for revision of the criteria themselves?

Questions for the Board of Review

The major purpose of the Guidelines is to provide you and the evaluators with enough relevant data to produce a comprehensive assessment of the programs.

1. How well was this achieved?

Not at all achieved	Achieved very little	Somewhat achieved	Achieved well	Achieved completely
1	2	3	4	5

2. How ambiguous were the data:

Not at all ambiguous	Not very ambiguous	Somewhat ambiguous	Fairly ambiguous	Completely ambiguous
1	2	3	4	5

3. Was complete information provided?

4. Was there too much redundancy?

5. Did the Guidelines help you to be open minded and objective?

6. What *additional* instructions should be added to the Guidelines?

7. What portions of the Guidelines could be *deleted* or reduced?

8. What revisions are needed in the criteria?

9. Was there agreement among Board members, and between Board Members and evaluators on the criteria?

    Yes

    No

    Comment:

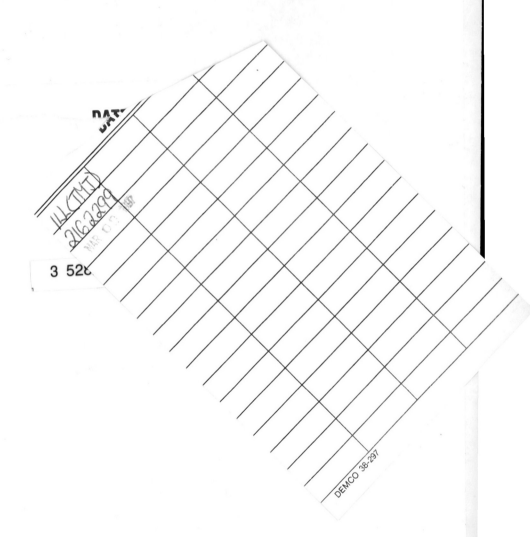

DEMCO 38-297